MW00928975

this journal belongs to

the brave compassionate
hardworking nurse
who is so tempted
to call-in-sick
but persisted to clock in
against all odds.

Cover Design by Duane Sue @Wellnessrush

Thank You!

for purchasing a copy of this awesome journal!

Inside you will find wealth of pages that you can use as a workbook, doodle pages, visual journal, track your health habits, gratitude, vision board, and so much more!

I hope and pray that this journal will aid you as you work on your self-care goals.

My mission is to help women like you find work life integration, thrive healthy in this busy world so you can live the life of your dreams.

Check out my website at wellnessrush.com for more wellness productivity tips.

Much love,
Duane Sue

Self care - is when you make time to make yourself whole to be able to serve God & others better.

-Duane Sue

MY LIFE GOALS

WELLBEING

RELATIONSHIP

CAREER/EDUCATION

MONEY

BUCKETLIST

MY PRIORITY IN CHECK

IMPORTANT-STAT	IMPORTANT- NON STAT
NON IMPORTANT- STAT	NON IMPORTANT- NON STAT

MY WELLBEING IN CHECK

PHYSICAL NEEDS	PSYCHOLOGICAL NEEDS

SPIRITUAL NEEDS	EMOTIONAL NEEDS

What area/s in my life I need to work on?

Self care checklist

SELF CARE IDEAS

DAILY

1. devotional/journal
2. prayer/meditation
3. eat more plant-based
4. carry a water bottle
5. 5 min daily exercises
6. leave work at work

WEEKLY

1. go out in nature
2. go to church
3. go for a walk
4. spend time w/ family/friends
5. get a massage
6. read a book

MONTHLY

1. go for a short road trip
2. visit a friend/family
3. check out a new place in town
4. go on a special date
5. do a fun activity with someone

YEARLY

1. vacation
2. retreat
3. long road trip
4. annual get together
5. declutter
6. annual health check

What do i need to start doing ?

date: _____________

3 things I'm thankful for	words to describe me today!

What's bothering you lately?

What are your "WHYS" in choosing healthcare industry as your career?

Write the words and phrases you need to hear right now?

How do you feel right now?

Write 6 survival strategies you regularly use during a stressful shift?

date: _____________

3 things I'm thankful for	words to describe me today!

How's your day beautiful?

If my body could talk to me right now, it would say…

"There's only one thing you can control - yourself"

-Duane Sue

What's bothering you lately?

What's your "go-to" self-care activity after a long exhausting shift?

How did you manage to overcome your challenges this week?

date: _____________

3 things I'm thankful for	words to describe me today!

If you could treat yourself today, what would it be?

Write down and deposit all your worries here this week.

How do you describe yourself right now?

How do you handle your difficult co-workers?

What gives you energy during long shifts? Look around you, what are you thankful for?

date: ____________

3 things I'm thankful for	words to describe me today!

What are the things that made you smile today?

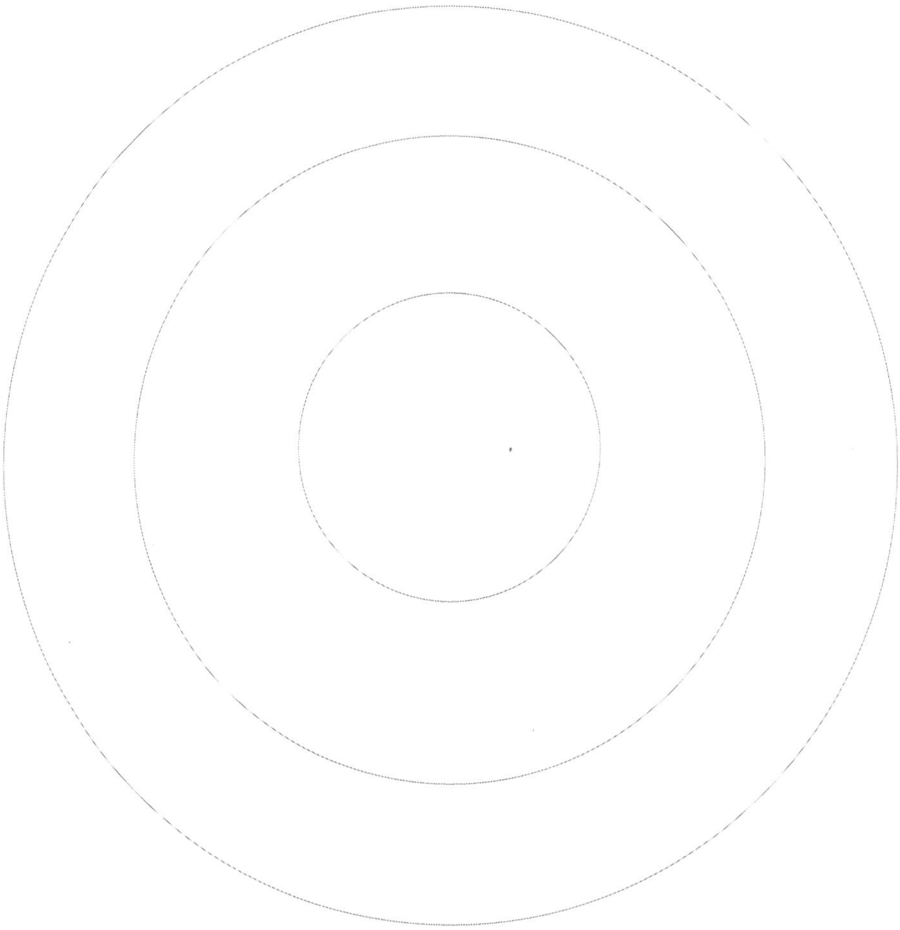

doodle away

draw lines, shapes, squiggles etc. inside the shapes.

List 5 things that are in your thoughts right now.

What are you looking forward to next week? Why?

Write down 3 things around you right now that make you happy? Why?

If someone will ask you right now, how are you doing? What would you say?

date: _____________

3 things I'm thankful for	words to describe me today!

If you have $20 in your hand right now, what would you do with it? Why?

Here's a brain dump- list the first 30 words you have in mind

Write an encouragement letter to yourself

What would make your life better today? Why?

Describe your emotions right now in words.

date: _____________

3 things I'm thankful for	words to describe me today!

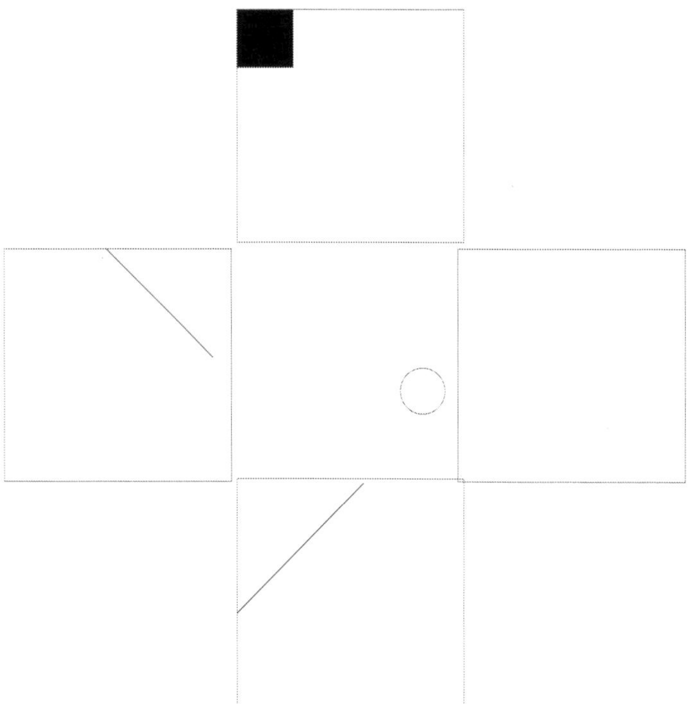

doodle away

draw lines, shapes, squiggles etc. inside the shapes.

How do you manage to face a patient/client when you are having a bad day?

What do you like most when helping patients/clients?

Write 3 things you are thankful for, and why?

Write the words and phrases you need to hear right now?

How do you feel right now?

How's your day beautiful?

date: ____________

3 things I'm thankful for	words to describe me today!

If my body could talk to me right now, it would say...

What's bothering you lately?

How did you manage to overcome your challenges this week?

If you could treat yourself today, what would it be?

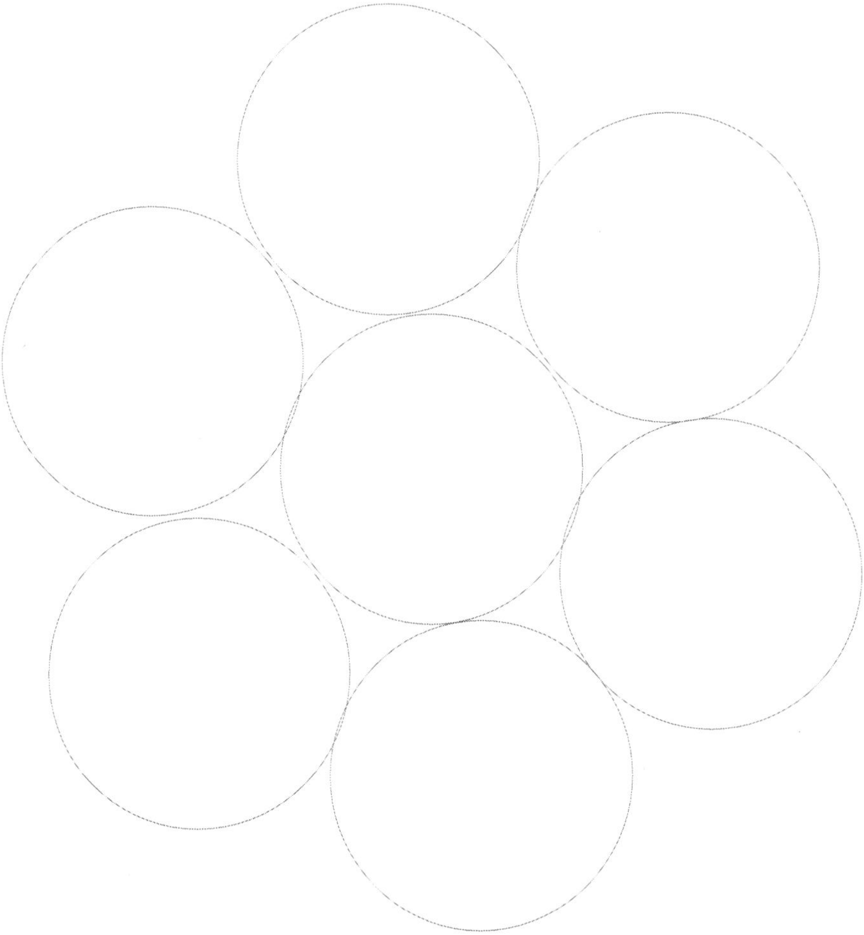

doodle away

write lines, shapes, squiggles inside the circles

How do you describe yourself right now?

date: _____________

3 things I'm thankful for	words to describe me today!

Look around you, what are you thankful for?

What are the things that made you smile today?

List 5 things that are in your thoughts right now.

What are you looking forward to next week? Why?

Write down 3 things around you right now that make you happy? Why?

date: _____________

3 things I'm thankful for	words to describe me today!

If someone will ask you right now, how are you doing? What would you say?

If you have $20 in your hand right now, what would you do with it? Why?

Here's a brain dump- list the first 30 words you have in mind

"Remember you are special and have unique capabilities to share to the world. Keep your candle burning."

-Duane Sue

Write an encouragement letter to yourself

What would make your life better today? Why?

date: _____________

3 things I'm thankful for	words to describe me today!

Describe your emotions right now in words.

Write 3 things you are thankful for, and why?

Write the words and phrases you need to hear right now?

How do you feel right now?

How's your day beautiful?

date: _____________

3 things I'm thankful for	words to describe me today!

If my body could talk to me right now, it would say...

What's bothering you lately?

How did you manage to overcome your challenges this week?

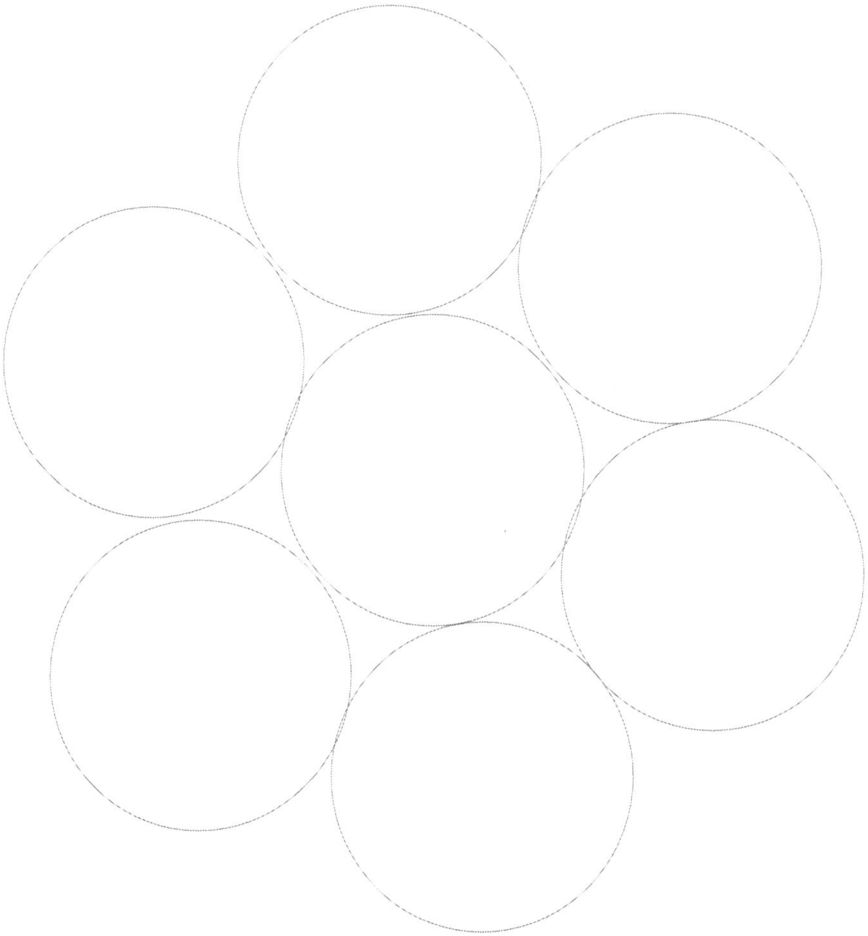

doodle away

write lines, shapes, squiggles inside the circles

If you could treat yourself today, what would it be?

How do you describe yourself right now?

VACATION
Planner

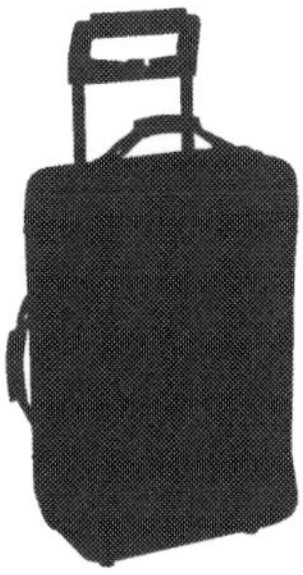

PACKING CHECKLIST

HOTELS AND TRANSPORTATION

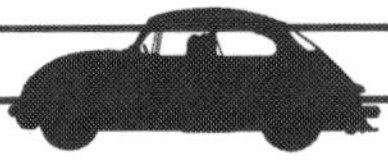

WHERE TO SHOP?

WHAT TO DO AND WHAT TO SEE?

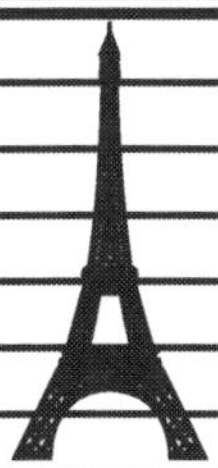

RECOMMENDATIONS AND NOTES

WHAT TO EAT?

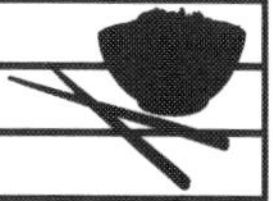

VACATION PLANNER

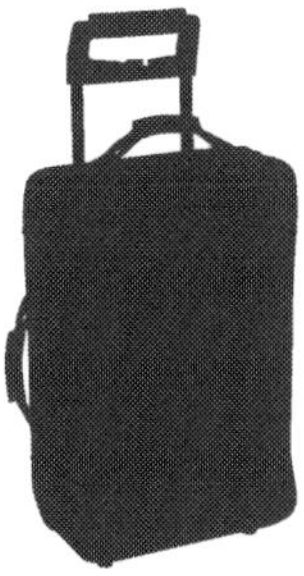

PACKING CHECKLIST

HOTELS AND TRANSPORTATION

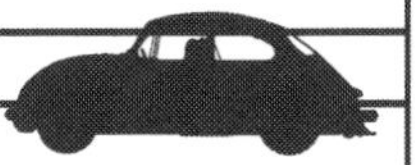

WHERE TO SHOP?

WHAT TO DO AND WHAT TO SEE?

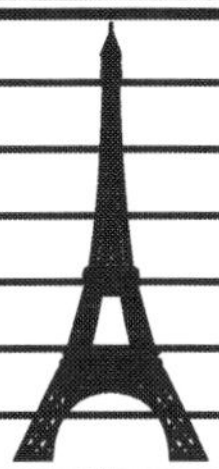

RECOMMENDATIONS AND NOTES

WHAT TO EAT?

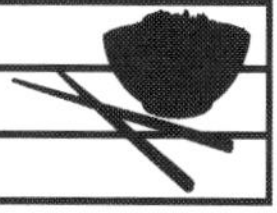

VACATION
Planner

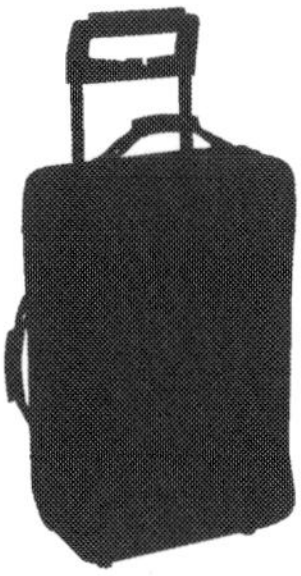

PACKING CHECKLIST

HOTELS AND TRANSPORTATION

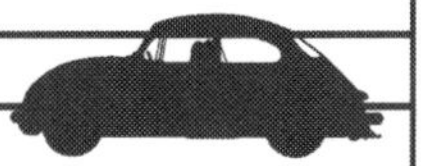

WHERE TO SHOP?

WHAT TO DO AND WHAT TO SEE?

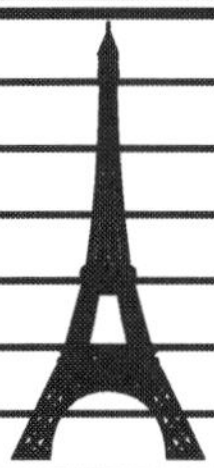

RECOMMENDATIONS AND NOTES

WHAT TO EAT?

VACATION
Planner

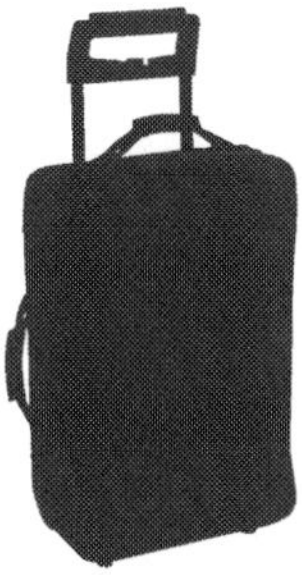

PACKING CHECKLIST

HOTELS AND TRANSPORTATION

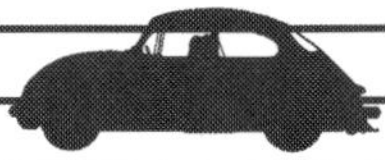

WHERE TO SHOP?

WHAT TO DO AND WHAT TO SEE?

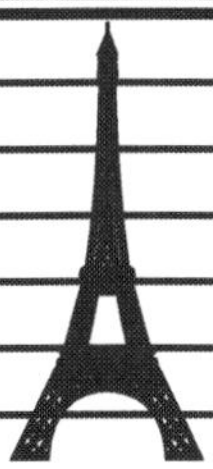

RECOMMENDATIONS AND NOTES

WHAT TO EAT?

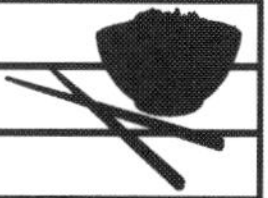

VACATION
Planner

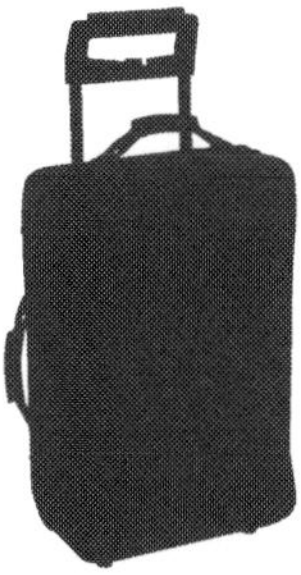

PACKING CHECKLIST

HOTELS AND TRANSPORTATION

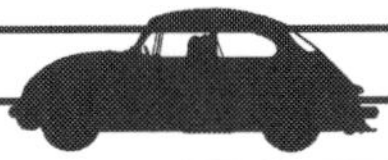

WHERE TO SHOP?

WHAT TO DO AND WHAT TO SEE?

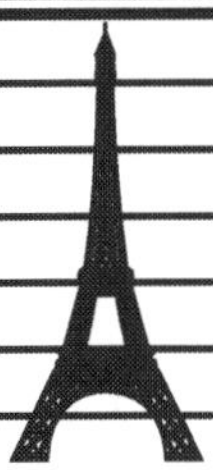

RECOMMENDATIONS AND NOTES

WHAT TO EAT?

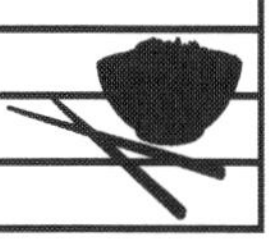

VACATION Planner

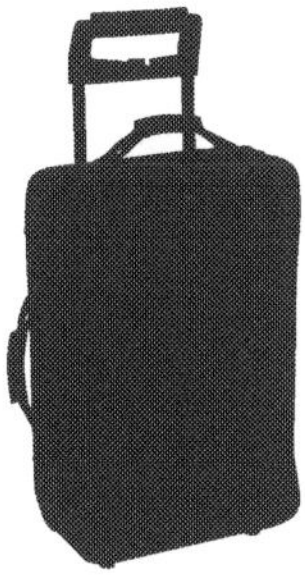

PACKING CHECKLIST

HOTELS AND TRANSPORTATION

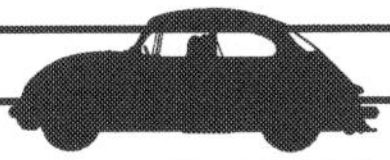

WHERE TO SHOP?

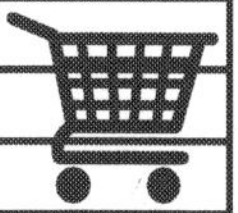

WHAT TO DO AND WHAT TO SEE?

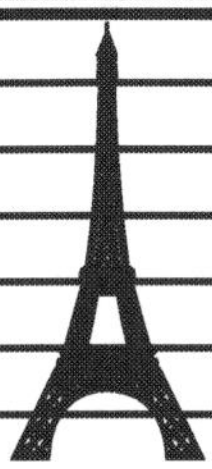

RECOMMENDATIONS AND NOTES

WHAT TO EAT?

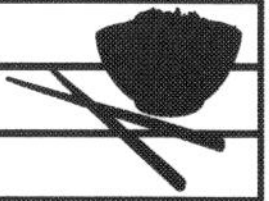

VACATION PLANNER

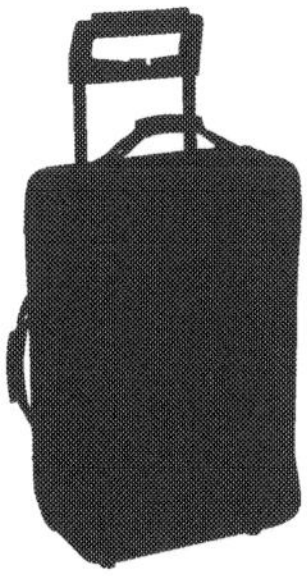

PACKING CHECKLIST

HOTELS AND TRANSPORTATION

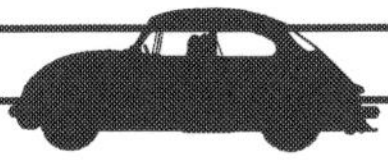

WHERE TO SHOP?

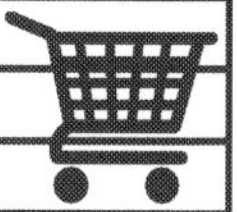

WHAT TO DO AND WHAT TO SEE?

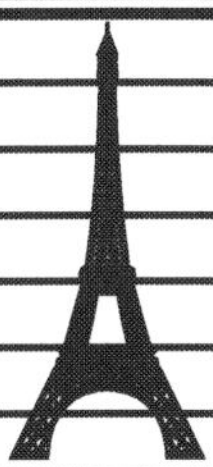

RECOMMENDATIONS AND NOTES

WHAT TO EAT?

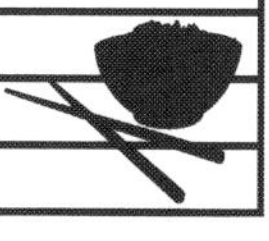

VACATION
PLANNER

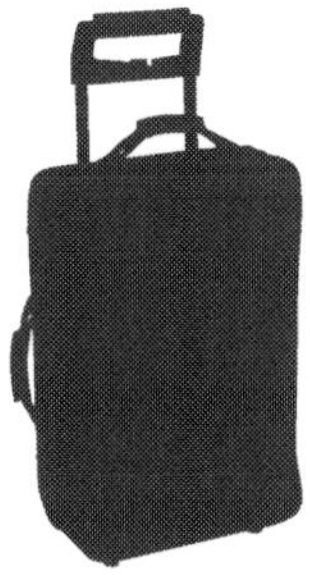

PACKING CHECKLIST

HOTELS AND TRANSPORTATION

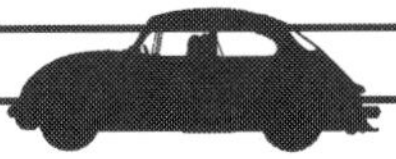

WHERE TO SHOP?

WHAT TO DO AND WHAT TO SEE?

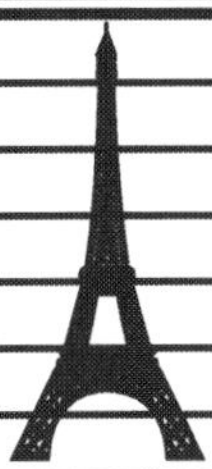

RECOMMENDATIONS AND NOTES

WHAT TO EAT?

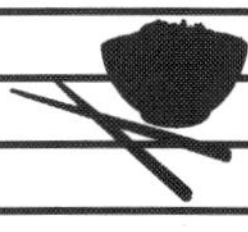

VACATION
PLANNER

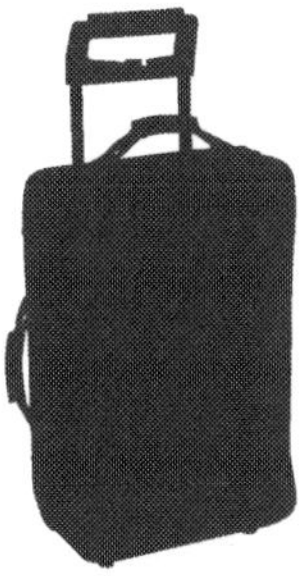

PACKING CHECKLIST

HOTELS AND TRANSPORTATION

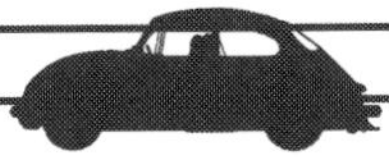

WHERE TO SHOP?

WHAT TO DO AND WHAT TO SEE?

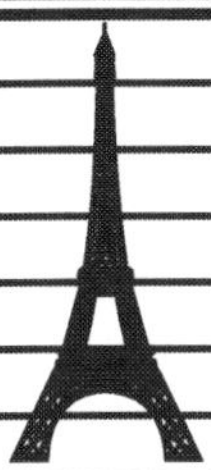

RECOMMENDATIONS AND NOTES

WHAT TO EAT?

VACATION
Planner

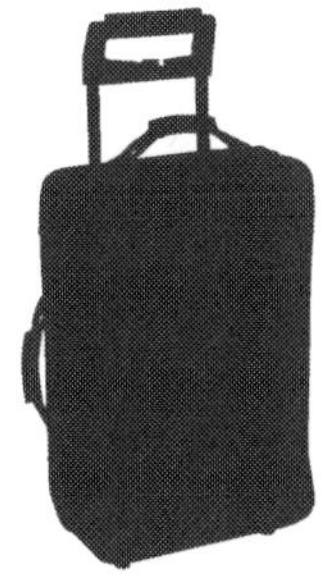

PACKING CHECKLIST

HOTELS AND TRANSPORTATION

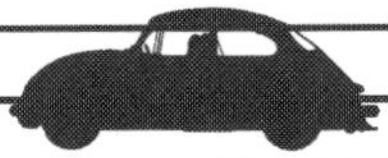

WHERE TO SHOP?

WHAT TO DO AND WHAT TO SEE?

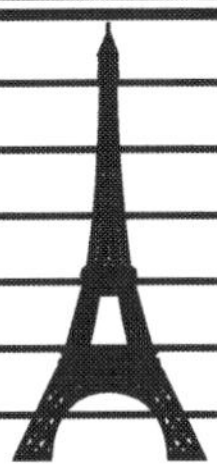

RECOMMENDATIONS AND NOTES

WHAT TO EAT?

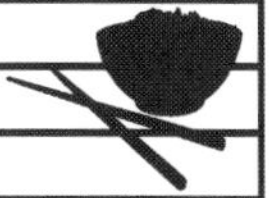

VACATION
PLANNER

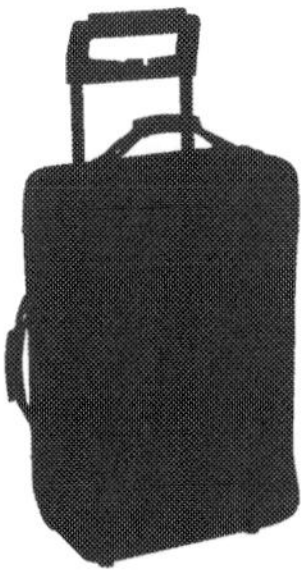

PACKING CHECKLIST

HOTELS AND TRANSPORTATION

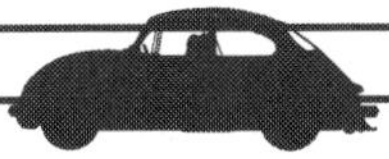

WHERE TO SHOP?

WHAT TO DO AND WHAT TO SEE?

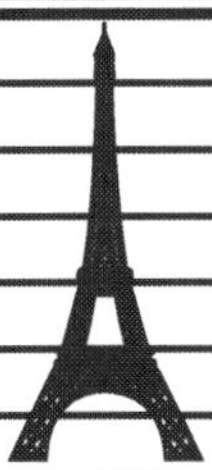

RECOMMENDATIONS AND NOTES

WHAT TO EAT?

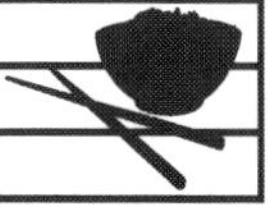

VACATION
Planner

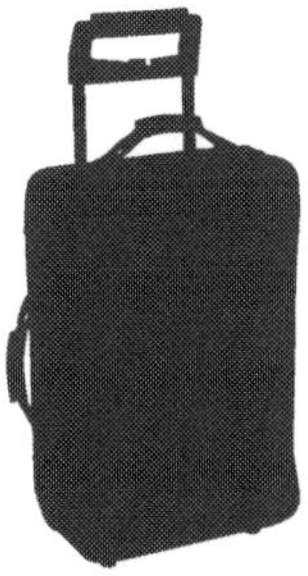

PACKING CHECKLIST

HOTELS AND TRANSPORTATION

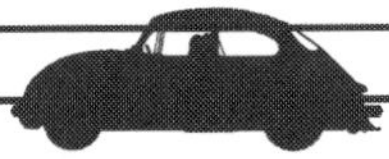

WHERE TO SHOP?

WHAT TO DO AND WHAT TO SEE?

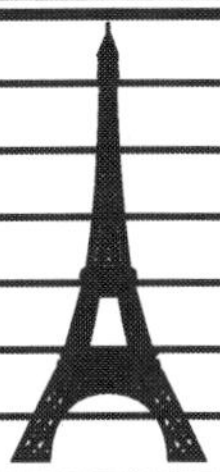

RECOMMENDATIONS AND NOTES

WHAT TO EAT?

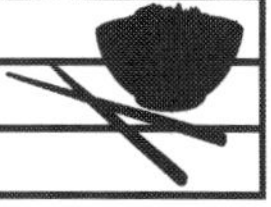

Healthy Self-care Tracker

IF YOU KEEP DOING IT, IT BECOMES PART OF YOU.

Month ____________

Year ____________

Day																
1																
2																
3																
4																
5																
6																
7																
8																
9																
10																
11																
12																
13																
14																
15																
16																
17																
18																
19																
20																
21																
22																
23																
24																
25																
26																
27																
28																
29																
30																
31																

Healthy Self-care Tracker

IF YOU KEEP DOING IT, IT BECOMES PART OF YOU.

Month ____________________

Year ____________________

Day																
1																
2																
3																
4																
5																
6																
7																
8																
9																
10																
11																
12																
13																
14																
15																
16																
17																
18																
19																
20																
21																
22																
23																
24																
25																
26																
27																
28																
29																
30																
31																

Healthy Self-care Tracker

IF YOU KEEP DOING IT, IT BECOMES PART OF YOU.

Month ____________

Year ____________

Day																
1																
2																
3																
4																
5																
6																
7																
8																
9																
10																
11																
12																
13																
14																
15																
16																
17																
18																
19																
20																
21																
22																
23																
24																
25																
26																
27																
28																
29																
30																
31																

Healthy Self-care Tracker

IF YOU KEEP DOING IT, IT BECOMES PART OF YOU.

Month ____________

Year ____________

Day																
1																
2																
3																
4																
5																
6																
7																
8																
9																
10																
11																
12																
13																
14																
15																
16																
17																
18																
19																
20																
21																
22																
23																
24																
25																
26																
27																
28																
29																
30																
31																

Healthy Self-care Tracker

IF YOU KEEP DOING IT, IT BECOMES PART OF YOU.

Month ____________

Year ____________

Day																
1																
2																
3																
4																
5																
6																
7																
8																
9																
10																
11																
12																
13																
14																
15																
16																
17																
18																
19																
20																
21																
22																
23																
24																
25																
26																
27																
28																
29																
30																
31																

Healthy Self-care Tracker

IF YOU KEEP DOING IT, IT BECOMES PART OF YOU.

Month ______________________

Year ______________________

Day																
1																
2																
3																
4																
5																
6																
7																
8																
9																
10																
11																
12																
13																
14																
15																
16																
17																
18																
19																
20																
21																
22																
23																
24																
25																
26																
27																
28																
29																
30																
31																

Healthy Self-care Tracker

IF YOU KEEP DOING IT, IT BECOMES PART OF YOU.

Month ____________________

Year ____________________

Day																
1																
2																
3																
4																
5																
6																
7																
8																
9																
10																
11																
12																
13																
14																
15																
16																
17																
18																
19																
20																
21																
22																
23																
24																
25																
26																
27																
28																
29																
30																
31																

Healthy Self-care Tracker

IF YOU KEEP DOING IT, IT BECOMES PART OF YOU.

Month ______________________

Year ______________________

Day																
1																
2																
3																
4																
5																
6																
7																
8																
9																
10																
11																
12																
13																
14																
15																
16																
17																
18																
19																
20																
21																
22																
23																
24																
25																
26																
27																
28																
29																
30																
31																

Healthy Self-care Tracker

IF YOU KEEP DOING IT, IT BECOMES PART OF YOU.

Month ______________

Year ______________

Day																
1																
2																
3																
4																
5																
6																
7																
8																
9																
10																
11																
12																
13																
14																
15																
16																
17																
18																
19																
20																
21																
22																
23																
24																
25																
26																
27																
28																
29																
30																
31																

Healthy Self-care Tracker

IF YOU KEEP DOING IT, IT BECOMES PART OF YOU.

Month ______________

Year ______________

Day																
1																
2																
3																
4																
5																
6																
7																
8																
9																
10																
11																
12																
13																
14																
15																
16																
17																
18																
19																
20																
21																
22																
23																
24																
25																
26																
27																
28																
29																
30																
31																

Healthy Self-care Tracker

IF YOU KEEP DOING IT, IT BECOMES PART OF YOU.

Month ______________________

Year ______________________

Day																
1																
2																
3																
4																
5																
6																
7																
8																
9																
10																
11																
12																
13																
14																
15																
16																
17																
18																
19																
20																
21																
22																
23																
24																
25																
26																
27																
28																
29																
30																
31																

Healthy Self-care Tracker

IF YOU KEEP DOING IT, IT BECOMES PART OF YOU.

Month ____________________

Year ____________________

Day																
1																
2																
3																
4																
5																
6																
7																
8																
9																
10																
11																
12																
13																
14																
15																
16																
17																
18																
19																
20																
21																
22																
23																
24																
25																
26																
27																
28																
29																
30																
31																

Made in the USA
Las Vegas, NV
03 December 2021

35951090R00106